FROM

TO RESTING

Joni Knapper

When you pass through the
waters, I will be with you; and
when you pass through the rivers,
they will not sweep over you…
For I am the Lord your God, the
Holy One of Israel, your Savior.
Isaiah 43:23

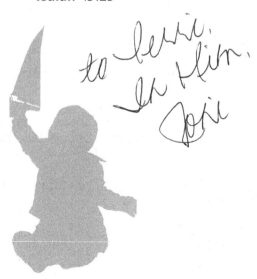

Surviving the Loss of My
Grandbaby, Saylor Irene

Printed in the United States of America

First Printing, 2023

ISBN 978-1-955791-70-0

Library of Congress Control Number: 2023917077

Ordering Information: Special discounts are available on quantity purchases by bookstores, corporations, associations, and others. For details, contact the publisher at sales@ braughlerbooks.com or at 937-58-BOOKS.

For questions or comments about this book, please write to info@braughlerbooks.com.

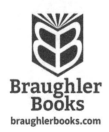

Braughler Books
braughlerbooks.com

2 Corinthians 1:3-5   Praise be to the God and Father of our Lord Jesus Christ, the Father of compassion and the God of all comfort, who comforts us in all our troubles, so that we can comfort those in any trouble with the comfort we ourselves receive from God. For just as we share abundantly in the sufferings of Christ, so also our comfort abounds through Christ. (NIV)

Contents

Foreword

I would like to take just a moment to provide a little background on the purpose of this memoir. When I initially started writing, it was in the form of a letter to Saylor Irene Scott, our fourth granddaughter. I started writing to Saylor when we received indicators that she may have a very short life expectancy. As time went by, the letter grew and I felt the Holy Spirit nudging me to share these thoughts with others who may be experiencing grief or infant loss.

I have been "a daughter of the King" and a Jesus follower since college. ("For those who are led by the Spirit of God are the children of God." Romans 8:14) My husband, Tim and I, have been married for 42 years and have three daughters, three "sons in love" and four granddaughters. Saylor, our fourth granddaughter, is the subject of this memoir, and you will learn more about her and our family as I share this story of how we loved her and lost her. It is not an easy story to tell or to read, but it is an important story that brings healing as I write. I pray whatever circumstances lead you to pick up this book, you will feel the deep love of the Father as you read it- and that you will also experience healing. I have utilized God's word in his holy Bible. Different translations have been studied and every effort has been made to accurately represent God and His word.

For a little background about us, Tim and I struggled with infertility and eventually welcomed our first child after about five years of infertility treatment. Due to our personal history of infertility it was especially difficult for us to watch our two younger daughters deal with the same issue. I came to recognize that our daughters' pain triggered in me all the hard and painful feelings that I had not totally recognized when we were experiencing our own difficult walk through infertility.

This seems a good time to advocate for healthy mental health. If there are issues that are causing you pain, please take some time to look at them, seek help from a professional, and do the hard work. I can attest to the fact that pretending and suppressing feelings are not helpful strategies. Unprocessed mental health difficulties are like physical wounds festering. Taking pain into the light of day is the beginning of good mental health.

I am a registered nurse and my background has been the neonatal intensive care unit (NICU), public health, home care and school nursing. I had no idea at the time how much my background was going to benefit my family as the years rolled by. In fact, as I look at my life, it is very clear to me that God was using past experiences to benefit my family and me, and also to allow a platform for me to build and grow. I have always LOVED being a nurse. It has been both an occupation and a ministry. Each new job built on the skills of the previous job, and He walked with me through the scary times and new positions in the field. ("For we are God's handiwork, created in Christ Jesus to do good works, which God prepared in advance for us to do." Ephesians 2:10)

The time period of Saylor's birth and life were toward the middle of the Covid-19 Pandemic that began in March 2020. As a result, we were very cautious and protective of this sweet young family.

All three of my daughters love babies. They all played with dolls until almost embarrassing ages. They all looked forward to becoming wives and mothers. Now that all three girls have their devoted and loving husbands, we were sure many more babies would be celebrated. It is still our great hope and prayer that more babies will come in the future, but it is important to say here that one life does NOT replace another. Having a "rainbow baby" (a term used to define a healthy baby after an infant or pregnancy loss) does not erase the pain of the baby who was lost. I do believe having more children will be part of the healing, but the pain will remain. One good friend who lost an infant said, "You never laugh quite as heartily again, and you are always closer to tears."

Well said, my friend. In short, losing baby Saylor has changed us. I only held Saylor in my arms for a few short months but she taught me so much. I learned about the sanctity, value and fragility of life. I learned to look deep into Saylor's eyes and allow her to communicate with me. She couldn't smile, coo, or move like other infants, but she could still communicate. I learned patience with special needs individuals. Saylor taught me to be kind, accepting, and less judgemental. She taught me to be present in the moment. Only God knows what the future holds, so live every moment of every day! Now that Saylor is in heaven with her Creator, I am even more excited about eternity. Her final gift to me was hope and faith in our heavenly reunion.

Our prayer throughout this journey has always been that God would be glorified. We have prayed for others to come to know Jesus in a personal relationship because of this story. We have hoped through our tears that someone may be watching how tenderly Saylor was loved and cared for during her short time with us. Saylor's life matters: She was here; She was loved; and her life made a difference. And we will never be the same. Thank you for walking part of this journey with us.

Two additional purposes for this memoir are comfort and peace for other grieving families and an increased awareness of Krabbe Disease and other chromosomal abnormalities.

My deepest thanks and admiration go to Saylor's mama and dada, Betsy and Evan Scott. This is *their* precious child and *their* story. I appreciate them allowing me into the sacred space of their young family. They graciously shared Saylor with me and I am forever grateful.

Thank you's to the following healthcare workers who touched Saylor's life:

Dr. Greg Utter, perinatologist, Dr. Marcia Johnson, obstetrician, Dr. Anthony Tackman and Dr. Robin Pierucchi, neonatologists, Dr. Maria Escolar, Pittsburgh Children's Hospital, Bronson Methodist Hospital NICU staff, Dr. Amie Simpson, Dr. Renee Lassila, and Dr. Sherry Pejka, pediatricians, Dr. Robert Simon, Internist and Emergency Medicine; and our visiting homecare nurse, Linda Hibst, RN. We could not have walked this path without the expertise, professionalism and compassion of Saylor's team.

I want to share my appreciation for editing help from two friends, Carolyn Massey and Penny Briscoe.

Additional thanks to Mike Miller, GraceSpring Bible Church; my Bible study friends, Pastor Rob and Sandy Cook; and our wonderful families and friends who walked this journey with us. I especially want to thank our other three grandchildren, Emma, Nora, and Leia, who deeply loved their first cousin and are also grieving this big loss in their young lives. Thanks also to our other daughters and their husbands, Steph and David and Sara and Eric. Much love and appreciation to my husband, Tim, who patiently provided time and space for me to write.

While this story is about Saylor Irene Scott, it is also about Jesus Christ and how He walked with us during this journey. ("The heart of man plans his way, but the Lord establishes his steps." Proverbs 16:9)

From wrestling to resting is the name I landed on for this memoir and the reasons will be evident as you read. In the weeks and months while we were waiting for Saylor to be born, I WRESTLED with God. Capital letters wrestled. I prayed and begged and did everything within my power to convince God that Saylor deserved a miracle; that we deserved a miracle. God did provide a miracle, although it was not the one I wanted. The miracle that He gave us was His presence and comfort while we grieved. The Lord worked mightily in my heart as I was wrestling, but the big work happened when I stopped wrestling and started resting. Resting in His will and His power and His comfort.

I already mentioned that I dedicated my life to the Lord in college. I believe most of us know something about God. We have heard about Him and maybe even attended church or Sunday School. But, even Satan believes in God. Satan is very aware of God and His power. The Lord wants more from us than just belief. He seeks an intimate relationship with each one of us. My faith walk has been transformed from memorizing bible stories into falling in love with Jesus. It is about a relationship, not a religion. This story will demonstrate how my faith was transformed as I learned to rest with the Savior while we said goodbye to our granddaughter.

Chapter 1

Answered Prayers

"For you formed my inward parts; you knitted me together in my mother's womb. " Psalm 139:13

We have loved vacationing in Florida all of our lives. Early in our marriage, my parents purchased a condominium on the beaches of Sanibel in Florida and the fun series of vacations began. From a young, newly married couple in 1980, to a young couple with a family, we visited this retreat at least once a year. The warm sunshine and condo on the beach became a place of respite from our busy lives. As a result, our children grew up on the Gulf of Mexico, playing in the warm surf and sand. The southwest Florida beaches became our happy spot.

In early March of 2021, our middle daughter, Betsy, and her husband Evan joined us on a Florida vacation and shared the wonderful news that they were pregnant. This baby was so deeply wanted and loved and we were all so thrilled. Betsy and Evan had experienced two previous miscarriages and had been trying again to conceive a baby for over a year, so we were nervous - but trusting that this baby would be born alive and well.

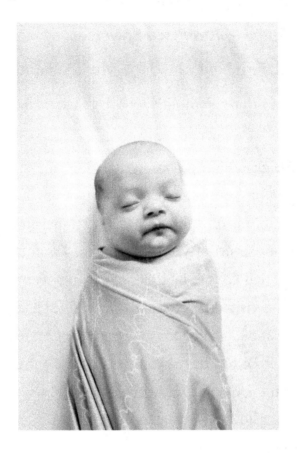

As the pregnancy progressed, all signs looked good. Progesterone and HCG levels were encouraging. Happily, Betsy and I took some time to visit our favorite children's store in Naples to buy a little pink and a little blue. We were so excited to finally be able to do this, and I will never forget this special outing with my daughter. There are times in all mom's hearts when we look forward to special occasions such as wedding days and welcoming children.

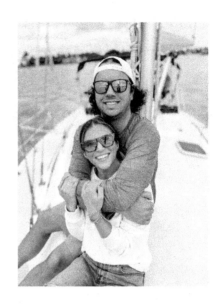

My husband and I hosted a gender reveal at our home in Michigan on May 2nd. Betsy was 13 weeks pregnant. The three granddaughters were part of the reveal and they used pink and purple paint in water guns to announce to their doting families and other guests that this precious bundle was a baby girl. Betsy and Evan had on white clothing, and their nieces sprayed them while we all rejoiced in the exciting news. The cousins were so excited to welcome their first cousin and forever playmate.

I have never seen our daughter or her husband as happy as they looked that day. There was good reason for their joy as the initial scan for common birth disorders was negative and we had no reason to suspect anything but a beautiful, bouncing, baby girl.

Mother's Day would follow and it was such a blessing for Betsy to celebrate for the first time ever, being a mama. Morning sickness and fatigue followed, but the joyful parents never complained and were filled with hopeful anticipation. The previous miscarriages cast only a shadow, and we were all very hopeful and excited. Clearly, this baby was already deeply loved and cherished.

Chapter 2

Pregnant and Loving It

"Before I formed you in the womb I knew you, and before you were born I consecrated you."

Jeremiah 1:5

Betsy and Evan were so thrilled to be pregnant. Much intentional time was spent preparing their new home for Baby Saylor. The nursery was decorated in pink and white. MANY hours were spent trying to hang the wallpaper, and eventually the room was ready. Because Saylor has three older girl cousins, Saylor already had a full closet of hand-me-downs. Clothes were organized by size and season, books were arranged near the rocking chair - and the bathroom showed off towels, washcloths and a baby tub.

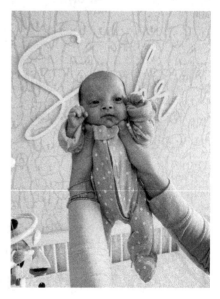

All of my sisters threw a beautiful baby shower for Betsy and Saylor in August. They received lovely gifts, and everyone was getting very excited to meet young Miss Saylor. My sister, Jane, had her home dressed up in pink to welcome this sweet child. The day of the shower was a very joyous one that we would later look back on to reminisce about happier days. It was nice to have a fun memory of "normalcy" before our worlds fell apart.

Evan spent his evenings reading books to the unborn Saylor. As I mentioned, Betsy had lots of nausea and vomiting but was a good sport about it, especially as she had waited so long for this pregnancy. The summer happily passed nearby at our Gull Lake cottage where Betsy and Saylor floated on our paddle board while Evan gave them rides around the dock. Both joyful parents felt Saylor's kicks and movements and often listened in awe to her heartbeat. There were boat rides, picnics, and sunning in Betsy and Evan's new backyard. The timing was perfect as Betsy and Evan had purchased their first home in February.

Saylor's name has great significance. My family has generations of sailors, sea captains, and sailboat racers. In fact, racing sailboats is one hobby my husband and I share. Changing the spelling to Saylor made her name more unique, and her parents loved the sound of SAYLOR SCOTT. Her middle name, IRENE, was Evan's grandmother's name and also the name of Betsy's great-grandmother. Saylor already had two of her namesakes in heaven praying for her.

Chapter 3

Ultrasound Horror

"For God gave us a spirit not of fear but of power and love and self control." 2 Timothy 1:7

After the 20- week anatomy scan, the kids left heartsick. Their world and ours had just been turned upside down. They had anticipated beautiful visions of their sweet baby. Instead, they were told the baby was very small and had no stomach and no kidneys. I will never forget this phone call. We were all devastated.

Betsy was referred to Maternal Fetal Medicine - and we were all so very concerned. But we continued to trust God and pray that this precious baby girl was going to be fine.

Maternal Fetal Medicine, MFM, turned out to be a huge blessing, and, specifically, their doctor, Greg Utter, was a gift. It was confirmed that Saylor was very small for gestational age, but they did locate her stomach and a single horseshoe kidney. Ultimately, after multiple scans, Dr. Utter recommended an amniocentesis so they could know how to be prepared at her birth.

Weeks later, sometime in August, we were told that Saylor had Deletion of the First Chromosome. Although shocked, we knew that Evan has a half-brother who had been diagnosed with Deletion of the First Chromosome. However, there were no indications that Evan carried this gene, so we were not prepared to hear this news. Later, though, we learned that it was possible to carry the gene but be perfectly healthy as in Evan's case.

A few days later we received even worse news. Dr. Utter told Betsy and Evan that Saylor also had an abnormality of the 14th Chromosome, which leads to Krabbe Disease, a form of Leukodystrophy. This disease is a progressive neurological condition which causes severe neurological damage and eventual death. The best case scenario, we were told, was that we might be blessed with our sweet Saylor for only two years.

Because both of these conditions are so rare, few people knew anything about either, and no medical experts we consulted had seen a baby with both. We were devastated! Would our precious girl live until delivery, die during or shortly after delivery, or die within a couple of years of her birth? These were all horrific options.

As believers in Jesus Christ, we did the only thing we knew to do, and that was to pray for healing and comfort. As we prayed, we also spent very intentional and valuable time with Baby Saylor, and one warm summer evening we recorded her heartbeat. I will never forget the sight of all 11 of our extended family, including the grandchildren, quietly and reverently listening to the strong and steady sounds of Saylor's heartbeat. We read her stories and talked to her as we patted Betsy's baby bump. We were not sure if we would have time with Saylor after she was born, so we tried to spend as much time with Betsy and Evan as possible.

I remember another summer evening when I read Saylor a few children's stories, not sure if I would have that experience with her after birth. Every moment we spent with Saylor in utero was a sacred and special time. We knew she could hear us and feel the love, so we did not waste any time without touching Betsy's baby bump and talking with sweet Saylor. We were determined that Saylor would know us, and, more importantly, know how deeply she was loved and cherished. Our other grandchildren, Emma, Nora, and Leia, would continually ask Saylor's parents, "How is Saylor?" They were so very excited to meet their first cousin, and Betsy and Evan were very generous with their time. They patiently let all of us talk and interact with their sweet Saylor.

("If any of you lacks wisdom, let him ask God, who gives generously to all without reproach, and it will be given to him. But let him ask in faith, with no doubting, for the one who doubts is like a wave of the sea that is driven and tossed by the wind." James 1:6)

Chapter 4

Sacred Delivery

"This is the day the Lord has made; we will rejoice

and be glad in it." Psalm 118:24

The maternal fetal medicine physician, Dr. Utter recommended an early delivery at 37 weeks as babies with chromosomal issues can also have placenta issues. So on October 20, 2021, Betsy was induced for delivery. Due to Covid, she was allowed only two support persons, which were, of course, her husband, Evan, and me, her mother. I was so honored to be there. An additional blessing is that our oldest daughter, Stephanie, is a certified doula and also attended as part of the medical team.

Another complication (soon remedied) was the discovery that Saylor was in a breech position. Betsy visited a chiropractor who had good skill in getting babies to flip, so for several weeks we weren't sure whether Saylor was head down or if Betsy would need a Cesarean Section. Eventually on ultrasound, Baby Saylor was shown to be head down, so her birth plan was put into place mid morning on October 20.

Saylor's birth on October 21, 2021, at 3:08 a.m. was the most sacred and beautiful moment of our lives. We had a "Jesus" song list playing and battery operated candles in the delivery room. Saylor was born feisty with an Apgar Score of 8/10 and 9/10, weighing 4 lbs. 1 oz. In addition to the four of us in the room, there were seven people from the NICU, three labor and delivery nurses, and a physician. God was there, too! Saylor was delivered with a placenta that was starting to separate (placenta abruptio) and was only discovered during delivery. This event can cause stillbirth or serious issues after delivery, including blood loss and possible organ failure for the mother. Her placenta was within minutes of separating, the doctor thought, which would have

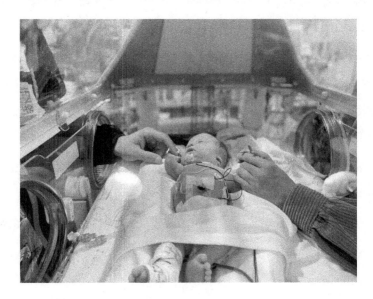

been catastrophic for both Saylor and Betsy. One of our first miracles, Saylor had survived birth and was in better condition than we had been prepared for. Praise God! Our new arrival impressed the doctors, and many of the staff commented on our faith and the sacredness of her birth. Our prayer was that this pregnancy, delivery, and baby would point to the power of Jesus – and it did.

But Saylor wasn't out of the woods yet. She had some difficulty breathing, so she was transferred to the NICU and put on oxygen and a CPAP (Continuous Positive Airway Pressure) with tube feedings. While in the NICU, doctors told us that Saylor was likely the only baby on the planet with these two chromosomal issues.

We had several amazing conversations with staff who fell in love with Saylor and whose lives were changed by her birth. Dr. Robin Pierucchi (a neonatologist) had spoken with us prior to Saylor's birth, and I remember her telling us that her desire was to

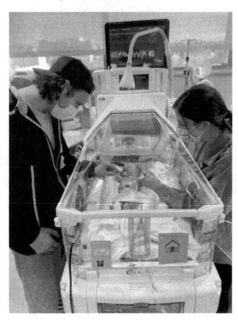

have Saylor tell us what Saylor needed. I loved how reverently she spoke of Saylor's life, and it comforted our souls. Later, after delivery, Dr. Anthony Tackman (neonatologist) came to Betsy's hospital room and said, "I have fallen in love with your daughter and she deserves a chance."

That conversation led to her treatment plan in the hospital and offered us much comfort. To the medical and nursing team who provided such tender and competent care, thank you seems inadequate.

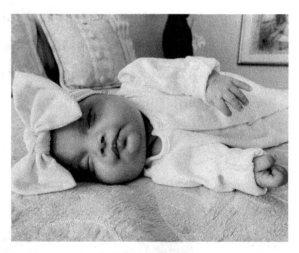

We were genuinely grateful for the competent, loving care they provided to baby Saylor, and her family. On October 29, eight days after birth, Saylor was discharged and finally home with her family.

Saylor was truly a beautiful baby. She had some soft dark curls and looked so much like her daddy, Evan.

She had big eyes, and even though we were told she was likely vision and hearing impaired, she followed her mama and daddy and turned toward their voices. Her ears looked "abnormal" but we found them adorable. Saylor was tiny, four pounds at 37 weeks gestation and only 15.7 inches long. Preemie clothes fit her well for the first couple months of her life. She had cute little hands that were usually held in a fist position and her tiny little feet were mostly still. She was a perfectly proportioned, petite little baby girl, and we adored her.

Chapter 5

Welcome Home

"For this child we prayed and the Lord has granted me my petition." 1 Samuel 1:27

The day Saylor came home from the hospital was a joyous celebration. The little family was so thrilled to be home all together. The front door was decorated with "It's a Girl" signs, and the entire neighborhood knew their baby had arrived. Saylor's tube feedings and apnea monitor complicated her care. At this point Saylor would breastfeed but couldn't eat enough to meet her caloric needs. She was also on several medications, including an antibiotic to prevent urinary tract infections as a result of her horseshoe kidney. God had directed my path to assist with Saylor's home care and provided a NICU background some 40 years previous when I worked as a new graduate in the very same unit that later cared for my granddaughter. He thinks of every detail and nothing escapes His hands - another miracle for which to thank God.

Saylor was able to enjoy her beautiful pink nursery that had been so lovingly prepared by her parents. She had the family heirloom baby bassinet in her parents' bedroom, in addition to her crib in the nursery. We knew Saylor was going to be small, so we had a few preemie outfits in which she looked just precious.

There is nothing like a baby to make a house feel like a home. Every detail revolved around sweet Saylor. God had provided a large master bedroom in this house, and the space was dedicated to this baby and her care. Partially because time together would be short, the little family wanted to be together as much as possible. One parent could sleep, while the other cared for Saylor. Occasionally, when I was there, both parents slept while Saylor and I ventured into the other rooms of their house. We would rock in the nursery, pace the floors of their downstairs living area, and a couple of times ventured out into the neighborhood in her baby buggy.

Chapter 6

Pennsylvania Children's Hospital

"In your goodness o God, you provided for the

needy." Psalm 68:10

Shortly after her discharge home, we received a phone call from Dr. Maria Escolar at the University of Pittsburgh Children's Hospital who invited us for a consultation. After some due diligence, we learned that Dr. Escolar was the world's leading researcher of Krabbe disease. We had no idea she existed until she called us, which we believe was a direct answer to prayer. Here I want to thank Dr. Robert Simon, who assisted us in determining that Dr. Escolar was indeed the right professional to see. He had researched Dr. Escolar and contacted colleagues all around the country while we collectively put together a plan of care for Saylor.

As believers in Jesus Christ, we had been praying for healing for months! While at this time there is no treatment for deletion of the first chromosome, when we heard about Dr. Escolar and her world-renowned treatment for Krabbe, we had to wonder if this was part of the miracle for which we had been praying.

On November 9, 2021, we boarded a private plane to Pittsburgh, piloted by a dear family friend, Mike Miller, who graciously agreed to transport us. We had to travel by private plane to keep Saylor safe as she did not tolerate her car seat for an 8-hour drive. Evan, Saylor, Betsy, and I flew to Pittsburgh for a consultation with half a dozen doctors at the University of Pittsburgh Children's Hospital. We left home not knowing what might happen, but we were confident that God had opened doors through which we should obediently walk. We believed that baby Saylor deserved every chance at life, especially with the knowledge that no treatment would mean a very early death.

In Pittsburgh, Saylor went through many tests as the doctors evaluated her condition. Sadly, we were told Saylor was not a good candidate for the stem cell transplant procedure. The rare combination of the two chromosomal abnormalities made Saylor very fragile and an outlier for their treatment. So, after many tears, we left the Children's Hospital and eventually flew home the next day, again thanks to pilot Mike Miller. Looking back, it seems obvious that such an invasive treatment would have proven too much for her frail little body. We would never have had the three and a half precious months at home with her if we had moved forward with the procedure. So while we were incredibly disappointed that the treatment would not work, we were very grateful that Betsy, Evan and Saylor could enjoy the holidays at home. (" ...for God gave us a spirit not of fear, but of power and love and self control." 2 Timothy 1:7)

Even though we had received bad news in Pittsburgh, God sent several amazing people into our lives. As it turned out, all of our Uber drivers were believers. The intuitively kind man who drove us home after Saylor's final appointment even prayed with us - and it touched our hearts deeply. It became evident that Saylor was going home with us, and we were continuing to fight for her and pray for healing.

By early December, Saylor weighed 6 pounds and was off her apnea monitor. Home nursing visits had been discontinued, and she amazed us every day. We lived in a place that was scary, yet sacred, and at the time, I didn't think we were living in denial. We understood her prognosis and yet continued to fervently pray for a miracle - more miracles, as we had already seen many. We tried so hard to be positive and to live each day so we could squeeze as many beautiful moments as possible into her life. ("Do not be anxious about tomorrow, for tomorrow will be anxious for itself. Sufficient for the day is its own trouble." Matthew 6:34)

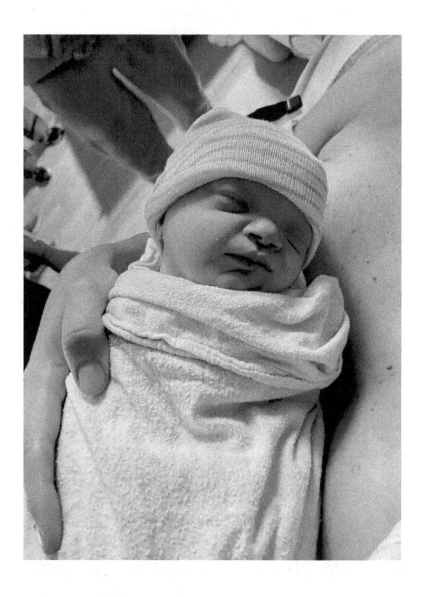

Chapter 7

Christmas 2021

"For a child is born to us, a son is given to us."

Isaiah 9:6

The holidays brought a special joy for our family as we celebrated the birth of Jesus along with the birth of Saylor. Attending services on Christmas Eve with Baby Saylor was a Holy event I will never forget. It was very emotional for me to watch Saylor in her parents' arms as we all worshiped the Christ child. I also observed many of our church family wanting to get a peak at this tiny baby they had been praying for, and yet respecting social distance with a fragile baby. Betsy would keep Saylor tightly wrapped to her body to minimize the friends who wanted to touch her. Evan was always close by, serving well the role of protective daddy. We were always concerned about disease exposure, especially because we were living in a time of high Covid pandemic infections. In fact, many extended family members were never able to meet Saylor because we were being so careful during the high respiratory virus season of winter.

Saylor was the center of Christmas for our family. We certainly hoped we would have more holidays with her, but we had no idea whether we would have another Christmas with her. I remember packing away the Christmas decorations in January and having a fleeting thought about how hard it would be to celebrate the next Christmas if we did not have her. Part of me was dreading the next Christmas for this very reason. And yet I trusted that our all loving God is always with us and "He has promised blessings after blastings". (Youssef)

Christmas is a favorite holiday for many, and that includes our daughter, Betsy. So, for God to bless them with Saylor for Christmas 2021 was an attribute of His to recognize the importance to this sweet little family. The Scotts were able to spend a quiet Christmas morning at home to celebrate Saylor's First Christmas, and later they joined the rest of our family for Christmas at our home. We all celebrated a little

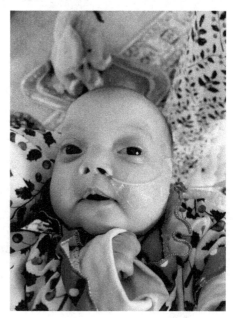

more tenderly that year, and while we celebrated the birth of Jesus, we also celebrated all the little miracles we had witnessed along the way.

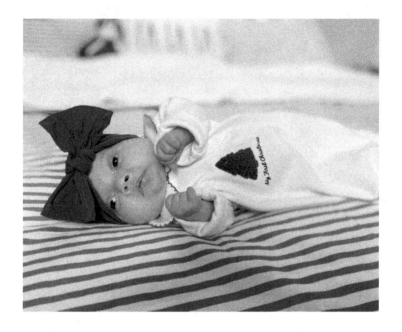

Chapter 8

'Florida Vacation

"For everything there is a season, and a time for every matter under heaven." Ecclesiastes 3:1

The Scott family wanted to take a family vacation with Saylor. We decided to visit Florida because my parents have a condominium where we could care for Saylor while still enjoying a family vacation. We stayed in Naples at my parents' condominium, which has so many wonderful memories for our children when they were growing up. Now, it is even more special because we have memories of Saylor there. Betsy and Evan lived in Tampa during their early married years so they really wanted to show Saylor the beautiful state of Florida. We introduced her to the pool, the Gulf of Mexico, bathing suits and warm sunny breezes. She even dipped her toes into the hottub, being held tightly in my arms as she wore her adorable bathing suits. We made many memories, the five of us. Chief (my husband's grandpa name) loved showing Saylor off - and we had some wonderful adventures. We returned to the children's shop in Naples

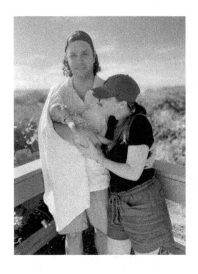

where her original outfits were purchased and bought Saylor something special for Easter. Saylor was living her best life!

Experience is the best educator, and life with Saylor taught me many things. One of the lessons I learned happened when we traveled by air with Baby Saylor to Florida from Michigan. I used my well-honed denial skills, but nevertheless I could still pick up on the judgemental looks we received from other travelers when we were flying with Saylor. Many people were nervous about flying during the Covid pandemic, even while healthy, so I could understand their concern over a tiny baby flying under such extreme circumstances.

I could see the looks. Curiosity, horror, judgment, and

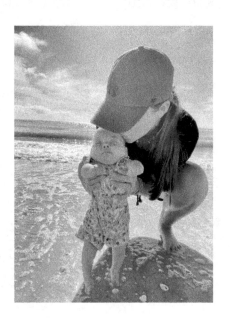

lots of sweet comments about how precious she was. One traveler even approached my son-in-law, Evan, and asked him if he was nervous about traveling during a pandemic with a small baby. Being a kind man he gently replied, "Yes, of course we worry. However, my daughter has a very short life expectancy, so we are willing to risk it in order to make memories with her." The traveler immediately felt sorry that she had said anything and I gave the stranger credit for putting into words what everyone else was thinking. I gave much credit to Evan, who was doing his very best to bless his daughter with wonderful memories in the short time they had her.

I learned much from Saylor in her very short life. One of those lessons was to be less judgemental. When making observations, remember that you don't know the whole story. It is often a good idea to give people the benefit of the doubt and not be quite so critical. As a mom, grandma, and registered nurse, I can see that I may have been one of these critical onlookers prior to this. Now I understand that these silent messages are hurtful and in our case contributed to more of the grief we were experiencing. It was a once-in-a-lifetime trip for this family with their precious daughter, and we didn't need the judgment or criticism from others who did not understand the situation.

Chapter 9

Back in the Hospital

"Behold, I am doing a new thing; now it springs forth, do you not perceive it? I will make a way in the wilderness and rivers in the desert."

Isaiah 43: 19

Shortly after our return from Florida, Saylor was admitted to the hospital with aspiration pneumonia. In fact, we were supposed to stay in Florida for several more days, but her parents felt we should return home early so Saylor could keep some scheduled appointments. Another miracle is that we were home when Saylor became sick. It would have been so difficult to hospitalize Saylor in a strange facility without any of our trusted medical team and family support. As I've said, Krabbe Disease and Deletion of the First Chromosome are both incredibly rare, and any unfamiliar healthcare professionals would have had a terrible time understanding our baby.

The day after our return, Saylor started having signs of respiratory distress. We went to the doctor, who made the decision to admit her to the hospital. Saylor was started on oxygen and spent several days on the pediatric floor. Despite our Florida trip, Saylor tested negative for respiratory viruses and the Doctors determined her symptoms were caused by an aspiration and had nothing to do with exposure while traveling. This was incredibly comforting to me as her "nurse" grandmother, and we were grateful that Saylor had not picked up a respiratory virus - or worse - while traveling.

When Saylor was hospitalized, her parents were very involved in her care. Saylor was never alone in the hospital. Both Besty and Evan stayed overnight while she was hospitalized. They changed diapers, helped with feedings, and held Saylor as often as they could. They received many compliments about how well they cared for Saylor, and the staff expressed their wishes that all children could have such attentive parents. Betsy and Evan were complimented but also incredulous at the idea that all parents wouldn't be just as devoted. Their hearts and their home were empty and sad when Saylor was not there, so the exhausted parents were thrilled when she was discharged to go home again. Saylor returned to their happy place on oxygen as she was not able to maintain her oxygenation levels. (While we were hoping to wean Saylor from the oxygen, in the end it was never to be.)

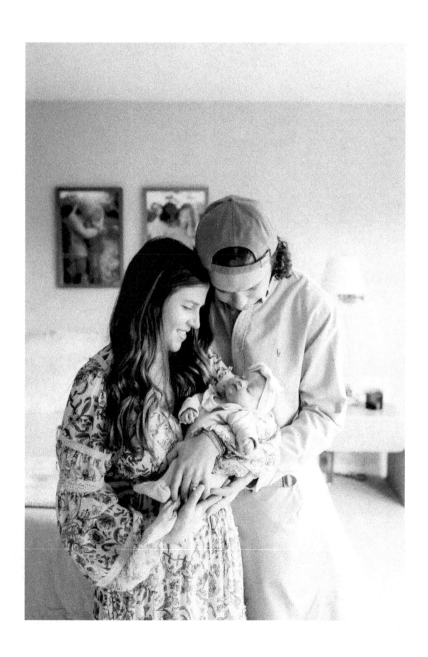

Chapter 10

My Sunrise Baby

"Let everything that has breath praise the Lord."

Psalm 150:6

I call baby Saylor my Sunrise Baby. I stayed the night for the first week they were home from the NICU and then occasionally just to offer support. Since I am a crack-of-dawn riser, it was easy for me to take the early morning shift so her tired parents could sleep. I would watch the sunrise with Baby Saylor and pray for her recovery and healing. It was a special time for just the two of us. I always knew I may not have the time with Saylor that I have had with my other grandchildren, so I spent as much time as I possibly could with the Scott family. I am sure the rest of my family felt my absence, but they patiently and lovingly did not complain. We all knew this was precious time.

I remember one of the last moments I was with Saylor; her parents had asked me to come stay with her so they could take a walk. It didn't surprise me when Betsy and Evan returned within 30 minutes of leaving because they missed her. I kidded them at the time, but I also totally understood their frantic desire to spend every possible moment with Saylor. Betsy told me she missed her - even in the 15 minutes it took to take a shower and get dressed. Evan and Betsy would fight jokingly over who had more time with her. While many parents are grateful for a break, they were soaking up every possible moment, even in their deep fatigue.

I also remember the last time I held Saylor alive; she just melted into my chest. This posture was very unlike Saylor who would usually arch her back and head away from whomever was holding her. (We were never quite sure why Saylor was more comfortable in this position but attributed it to her increasing GI distress.)

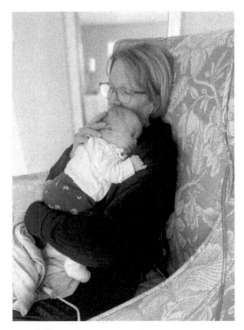

Betsy and I both commented on it and enjoyed the special snuggles. We were leaving for Florida the next day for trips with our other children. I said goodbye to Saylor, perhaps naively confident that she would be here when I returned from our trip. Unfortunately, that was not to be, and we returned to our lovely Saylor's grieving and heartbroken parents.

Chapter 11

Saylor's Shocking Death

"Weeping may tarry for the night, but joy comes
with the morning." Psalm 30: 5

In the early morning hours of February 5, Betsy and Evan found Saylor blue, cold and unresponsive. Despite this shocking find, they performed CPR, called 911, and watched in horror while paramedics were unsuccessful in reviving their darling daughter.

Though we knew our time with Saylor would be short, we were hoping that time would be measured in years, not just a few months. As a result, Saylor was not yet in hospice and her death at home needed to be investigated by law enforcement. The heavy grief and loss, were compounded by the Child Protective Services officials, search warrant, and required autopsy. Fortunately, the medical examiner did contact Betsy and Evan within a week to tell them he could determine from his examination that Saylor was well cared for and deeply loved. While that was reassuring, the wondering about what actually killed Saylor was tormenting us all - and three months of agony would follow before we knew the autopsy results. Finally, it was confirmed that Saylor died of complications from Krabbe Disease. In fact, instead of celebrating Saylor's six month birthday, we were hearing about the details of her autopsy report. As Krabbe Disease progressively attacks and destroys the myelin sheath of the nerves, it is believed her little brain simply forgot to breathe.

Our daughter, Betsy's sister Sara, and her husband came running to the sides of the Scott family during the tumultuous morning we lost Saylor. We were in Florida, and Sara and Eric were due to travel to meet us there - until the dreadful phone call. They graciously canceled their trip and were a tremendous help to all of us during the difficult time. Sara was working as a hospice social worker and thus was a huge help as Betsy and Evan were saying goodbye to Saylor. Tim and I flew home immediately and Steph, David and their family left Florida later that same day. I find it interesting and serendipitous that both of Bety's sisters were present, one at the beginning of Saylor's life and the other at the end.

Looking back I wonder if we should have started hospice sooner in order to avoid the trauma of how her home death was handled. I know hindsight is 20/20, but I add this as some advice for families who may be in a similar situation. It is never an easy decision to engage in hospice, but my experience has always been that they provide tremendous comfort and insight. And in this regard, I believe her passing would have been less traumatic for Saylor's parents and even the rest of the family. With an expected death, there would not have been an investigation, CPS, and search warrant. However, during our short time with Saylor, her parents stayed in touch with the University of Pittsburgh care team. We had asked the nurse practitioner about hospice, and they did not feel it was time, so I believe we all felt Saylor had more time with us.

I know Saylor was a tremendous fighter. We always commented on how active Saylor was prior to birth. From the prenatal kicks and rolls, she would show us that she was brave and strong. Despite that, after her birth occasionally she would show signs of neurological decline. For example, her eyes would roll back up into her head, her sucking reflex would deteriorate, and she could not smile. Although we were able to recognize "her smile". We could see her deep intent when we talked to her. And then there were days when she was absolutely terrific and looked very alert, which is how Saylor was the day before she died. Her visiting nurse,

Linda, had visited and thought she looked wonderful. Linda was as shocked as we were when we told her of Saylor's death.

("For I consider that the sufferings of this present time are not worth comparing with the glory that is to be revealed to us." Romans 8:18)

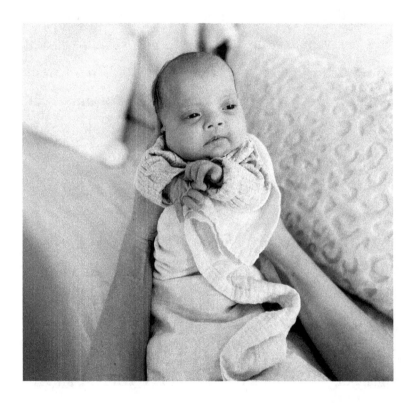

Chapter 12

Rockstar Parents

"For I can do everything through Christ who gives me strength." Philippians 4:13

I told Saylor while she was here with us that her mama and dada were extraordinary. They provided for her every need 24 hours a day, seven days a week for the months they had her. She was kissed, snuggled, sung to, danced with, swaddled, cuddled, prayed over, and dedicated to Jesus, every moment of her too short life.

Our son-in-law and daughter were superstars during Saylor's short life. Evan quickly learned how to change her NasoGastric tube, use the feeding pump and later the oxygen concentrator. Their master bedroom eventually became a mini hospital room and the epicenter of Saylor's care. They provided feedings every three hours, checked her oxygen saturation, administered medications and drove her to countless appointments. Betsy was pumping and using breast milk with some formula to supplement via tube feedings. So the every-three-hour feedings would take at least 40 minutes or so. While as Nana I was wondering how long they could keep this up, I knew Betsy and Evan loved every minute of the long hours and exhausting care of Saylor. There was no question they would happily return to those sleep deprived days just to have more time with their Saylor.

Added to the physical exhaustion, was the emotional turmoil. Actually, I believe the emotional weight was far heavier than the physical, watching for signs of improvement or deterioration, the anticipation of her premature passing, and the deep sadness we all felt as we grew closer to Saylor every moment of every day. It was an excruciating but sacred journey. Families who have lost children with Krabbe equate it to watching a freight train approach your child knowing there is nothing you can do to stop it. As a nurse, I thought I was seeing some signs of decline, but as a nana I remained extremely hopeful and confident that God would heal Saylor and we would somehow beat the odds. I was conflicted between hopeful optimism and preparatory reality. As sailors, we are used to evaluating the sky and weather conditions, prior to going out on the water. In fact this tumultuous time felt very much like the rolling sea and changing weather. The waves would increase some days, flatten on others, and we were constantly evaluating our baby. ("Suddenly a furious storm came up on the lake, so that the waves swept over the boat. But Jesus was sleeping. The disciples went and woke him, saying, "Lord, save us! We are going to drown!" He replied, "You of little faith, why are you so afraid? Then He got up and rebuked the winds and the waves, and it was completely calm." Matthew 8: 24-26)

I always knew Betsy and Evan were special people. I am a proud mama, of course, and at this point I had known Evan for about ten years. However, my respect and admiration grew daily as we watched the two of them navigate this great tragedy in their young marriage. Not only did they provide tender loving care for Saylor, but they have been trying so very hard to grieve well and move on for what God has next for them. "And the peace

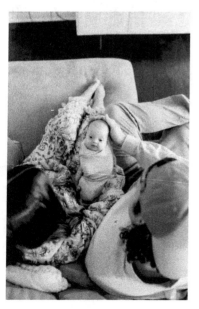

of God which surpasses all understanding, will guard your hearts and minds in Christ Jesus. " Philippians 4:7.

Because both carry the auto recessive genetic trait that leads to Krabbe, and Evan also carries the gene for deletion of the first chromosome, future pregnancies are risky without genetic testing. So their future children will need to be conceived via In Vitro Fertilization (IVF) or through adoption. This young couple was not only grieving their first born, but also future children. A very heavy load indeed for anyone to process, they became focused on completing their family. Saylor showed them how much they loved being parents. And they believe Saylor wants them to have more babies, although it is impossible to replace one child with another.

The deep grief over their loss will always be present, but I pray the intensity will be soothed a bit as they move forward and add on to their family. I am committed to making Saylor's memory a forever part of our family. Every year we will hang her stocking and fill her Easter basket. We will celebrate her birthday and the special gift she was and is to us. Saylor's life had a purpose and God had a plan.

Chapter 13

Surviving Without Saylor

"For my thoughts are not your thoughts, neither are your ways my ways, declares the Lord." Isaiah 55:8

In the days that followed Saylor's passing, Betsy and Evan lamented continually at how much they missed her - how much their hearts actually, physically, hurt. Their arms ached and Saylor's home felt way too empty and quiet. When I visited, it was painful but also bittersweet to see things had stayed the same since Saylor left for heaven. Even months later her baby seat was still on the table. Her bassinet sits empty in the master bedroom. Saylor's bedroom is quiet and a physical tribute to the beloved baby who should have been sleeping there. The car seat base remains in the backseat of the family car. The stroller is parked expectantly in the garage. Pictures of sweet Saylor are everywhere but they almost make the house feel emptier because we are forced to fill our present with her past.

It is excruciating to watch our precious children, Saylor's mommy and daddy, grieve the loss of their only child. It is equally difficult to grieve the loss of our cherished grandchild, Saylor, while providing strength and comfort for our children. It is a tenuous tightrope to walk as grieving grandparents and also parents of grieving children. I write this to other grandparents who may be walking this difficult road, and I truly feel like it may be the most difficult thing I have ever done. So, If you are walking this road, give yourself some grace and take care of yourself. It is a long road and emotional marathon. (Helpful resources are listed at the end of the book.)

I was fortunate to have other grieving grandmothers walk this journey with me. It is a sad community no one wants to need, but if you look around and are as fortunate as I was, others will come forward and reach out to offer comfort and tips on recovery.

Allow others into your pain. It really does help to hear about others' journeys and what they have done to recover, heal and move forward in life. While it is tempting to curl up and not leave the comfort of your bed or home, healing will come with some hard work. Saying that, I also totally endorse taking days to stay home and be introspective, as a balance is important. Another recommendation I have is to seek counseling from a qualified Christian counselor with experience treating grief.

One query that continues to be difficult is answering that question: "So how many grandchildren do you have?" I would say four and burst into tears. Or I would say four and not elaborate. I even said three a few times just to avoid the conversation. The truth is that we have lost our last four grandchildren to death. Betsy and Evan had two miscarriages before conceiving Saylor, and our youngest and her husband have lost a baby to miscarriage. We have had so much recent loss; yet our oldest daughter and her husband have three beautiful daughters whom we cherish.

Chapter 14

A Family for the Scotts

"He gives the barren woman a home, making her
the joyous mother of children. Praise the Lord!"

Psalm 113:9

While we were still grieving the loss of Saylor, Betsy and Evan started looking for ways to be parents. They began researching adoption agencies and IVF. Actually I do not believe the grieving will ever be totally over but, hopefully, the intensity of the sting will be soothed a bit. As I mentioned earlier in my writing, one child does not replace another. Saylor will forever be a part of our family, and her parents' deepest desire is that we continue to say her name and celebrate her life. Saylor will always be their first baby and first daughter, and she is the one who made them parents.

To honor Saylor and her parents, we recently established a student scholarship for graduating high school seniors pursuing healthcare or special education. Every spring when the winner is announced, we plan to share Saylor Irene Scott's name and a little bit about her. It is a small way to keep her memory alive. We have also become involved with the foundation, KrabbeConnect. Until Saylor was diagnosed, we had no idea what Krabbe was, or the devastating progression of this illness. Thankfully, there were wonderful people who supported us emotionally, and we knew we needed to learn more about their cause.

Chapter 15

KrabbeConnect Foundation, #curekrabbe

"Love bears all things, believes all things, hopes all
things, endures all things. Love never ends."

1 Corinthians 13:7-8

Six months after our devastating loss of Saylor,
we were invited to a KrabbeConnect gala, "A Million
Dreams". Betsy and Evan were encouraged to go, so my
oldest daughter and I accompanied them on this trip.
We prayed that the event would be a part of our journey
of healing, and we were so right!

It was held in Minneapolis, which isn't too bad a
drive from our home; so we headed off for Minnesota
with heavy but expectant hearts. At some point early in
our journey with Krabbe Disease, my son-in-law, Evan,
reached out to the originators of this foundation. He
ordered some #curekrabbe bracelets and a window sticker
for their car. Little did we know that this would begin
a relationship with the KrabbeConnect Foundation
(info@krabbeconnect.org). The Foundation founders,
Ann Rugari and Stacy Pike-Langenfeld, had both lost

their own children to this dreadful disease. Evan had e-mailed them now and then during Saylor's short life. Eventually, we had to share our sad news with them - that Saylor had lost her fight with Krabbe and Deletion of the First, but also that she had been fully healed and was now living with her Creator in heaven.

All of us were absolutely thrilled to be at the Fundraising Gala among other "Heroes" and their parents, families who had lost their heroes, and the many medical friends of Krabbe who work on treatments and a cure. The children affected with Krabbe are referred to as Heroes. It was heartbreaking but also encouraging to hear of others' losses and know we were not alone in our grief. We watched many generous people donate their resources to KrabbeConnect. We remain hopeful that someday we will find a cure.

In the meantime, it is important to introduce Krabbe testing to all routine newborn screening in ALL STATES as there are measures that can treat this terribly progressive neurological decline that can begin soon after birth. Currently there are only nine states which routinely test all newborns with a Krabbe blood test. They are GA, TN, KY, MO, IL, IN, OH, PA, and NY. Other states with active efforts to add Krabbe testing to Newborn Screening are OR, MN, IA, WI, VA, and NC. Krabbe Disease is hereditary and currently there are no cures. In Michigan during 2020, there were 104,074 births and 58 conditions routinely screened. However, there are procedures to slow down the disease and improve the quality of life for children with Krabbe disease. In honor of SAYLOR IRENE SCOTT we are joining others in promoting routine newborn screening in the state of Michigan.

Chapter 16

From Wrestling to Resting

"Now faith is the assurance of things hoped for, the conviction of things not seen."   Hebrews 11:1

When we learned of the issues our adored Baby Saylor was facing, we took them immediately to the feet of Jesus. Our church, GraceSpring Bible Church, rallied around us. They prayed over Betsy, Evan, and Saylor. The entire church and, later, the entire community prayed for healing. They prayed week after week. I am forever indebted to our brothers and sisters in Christ who faithfully stormed heaven on our behalf.

Our dear friends, Pastor Rob Cook and his wife Sandy, offered constant support and many prayers. In 2019 Rob married Betsy and Evan on a warm June afternoon. Rob visited their home in late 2021 after Saylor came home from the NICU to dedicate her to Jesus. Some two and a half years after their wedding, Rob presided over Saylor's celebration of life. The two events were different and yet the same. Obviously, their wedding was a joyous occasion when they asked Jesus to walk with them on this journey called marriage. Saylor's service was beautiful, too. I would love to say it was joyous, but, honestly, it was heart wrenching. Pastor Rob called this chapter in Betsy and Evan's lives, "Precious and Deeply Loved", and we asked Jesus to continue to walk with us all as we grieved. Saylor's tiny body lay in the heirloom family bassinet and her parents made the decision to have her cremated. We closed her service with "I Speak Jesus" by Charity Gayle, which was the same song playing in the delivery room when Saylor was born. It was important for us to "Speak Jesus" over her birth and her return to Jesus. We celebrated her heavenly healing, and we believed she was safe in Jesus' arms.

But I had so many other emotions as part of my deep grief. I was angry with God that He had not healed my irreplaceable granddaughter. I thought he had missed a great opportunity to show His power. I thought he had wasted all of our time while we fervently prayed. Notice all the "I" comments ... While Betsy was still pregnant I had literally been wrestling with God and BEGGING him to heal Saylor. I thought I knew what was best and couldn't find a reason why God had let me down. Shortly before her delivery I added fasting to my prayers, again certain that Jesus would hear and heal.

Finally, I started to understand something that may sound ridiculous to others. I finally understood that I was not God. I started to see His heart and His character. I began to see that God sees the whole picture, while I see only a tiny part of the story. It's as if I am looking through the thick fog and can barely make out objects. Jesus slowly began to demonstrate His truths. Jesus is in charge, not Joni. We don't get to decide who God is or how He moves. And In addition to healing Saylor, Jesus was healing me.

First, I felt deeply loved, and I could feel His grief regarding our grief. I could feel his anger with death that began in the Garden of Eden and has followed humanity through this sin-filled world. I was reminded that Jesus wept at the loss of his friend Lazarus. He wept at that death, even though He knew He was going to raise Lazarus from the dead. Jesus was fully man and fully God, and He understands our deepest emotions. ("The Word became flesh and blood and moved into the neighborhood." John 1:14 The Message)

I began to understand that God has a plan and He sees all things-past, present, and future. Maybe it was possible that Jesus had a plan for choosing to heal Saylor in heaven rather than here on earth. The Apostle Paul talked about how to live is Christ and to die is gain. (Philippians 1:21) In other words, as believers in Jesus, we really can't go wrong. We either get to live here with Christ in our hearts or we go immediately into the presence of Jesus in heaven. I found as long as I walk closely with Jesus, the agonizing grief is manageable. The pain will forever be a part of who we all are, but I believe God is using the pain and grief to draw us, and hopefully others, closer to Him.

It may sound like I am over rationalizing and/or over spiritualizing to make myself feel better. It's possible others do not know Jesus personally and that all of this sounds very strange to them. It is also possible that the church or Christians in general have hurt some people deeply over the years and as a result they do not trust this God. Occasionally, I hear people say the Christian faith is a "Crutch". Yes, Jesus is my crutch and I am not ashamed to say it. ("For I am not ashamed of the Gospel, for it is the power of God for salvation to everyone who believes ..." Romans 1:16)

After the loss of Saylor, I was very selective about where I went and who I chose to be around. I listened to Christian music and podcasts, attended my Bible study and in general found I was comforted by Jesus as I tried to stay near Him. I was feeling a little like Peter may have felt when Jesus called Peter out of the boat to walk on the water. As long as Peter kept his eyes on Jesus, he was fine. But the minute he looked away, Peter would sink into the waves. If I wasn't walking closely with my Savior, I would sink into the depths of grief and despair.

My deep desire in writing this personal memoir and making myself vulnerable is to point others to Jesus. I do not have the answers; only He does. I believe with my entire being that Jesus is real and He loves us all. Salvation is not about religion or church membership. Salvation is much simpler than that, but it involves action on the part of the individual. That action is to simply believe He alone is Lord and to ask for forgiveness for the personal sins that one has committed. Good works do not stamp a passport to heaven. "For all have sinned and fall short of the glory of God." Romans 3:23

I have gone from wrestling *with* God while demanding a healing for Saylor, to resting *in* God as He holds Saylor. I can tell you that the latter is a much more peaceful place to be. Wrestling with God is exhausting! Resting in Him is the best place to be, whether a person is on top of the world or living a difficult nightmare like I have been living. Jesus makes every day better, and none of us knows when we may be called home suddenly. We should not put off the decision to put faith in Jesus. Eternity, heaven and hell are very real. It is a personal choice where one will spend eternity. ("The Lord is not slow to fulfill His promise as some count slowness, but is patient toward you, not wishing that any should perish, but that all should reach repentance." 2 Peter 3:9.)

Thank you for reading my family's story. It has been healing for me to write and process the events of loving and losing Saylor Irene Scott. R.I.P. sweet Baby Saylor. I love the idea of her resting in peace, but even more I love the idea of her being "Raised in Power". Pastor Jacob Rodriguez from CityLight Church introduced me to this term in one of his writings.

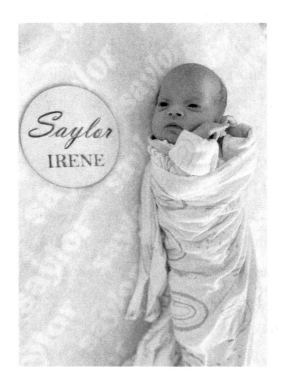

Saylor is not needing her earthly tent now. She has a new, healthy body; one free from chromosomal abnormalities, tubes, and pain. And Saylor is living her best eternity with Jesus, Krabbe free. I hope that you can meet her someday and I look forward to being reunited with my Sunrise Baby Granddaughter, and basking in the heavenly glow with my Savior.

May God bless all my readers with comfort, blessings and an eternity of peace with Jesus. "Beloved, I pray that all may go well with you and that you may be in good health, as it goes well with your soul." 3 John 1:2

A Note from Saylor's Mama:

Call it a mother's intuition but I knew something was wrong as early as 16 weeks pregnant. My belly was just so little that you could barely tell I was pregnant until about 30 weeks. I had a lot of close friends that were also pregnant at the time and I kept comparing my baby bump to their bumps and I barely looked pregnant compared to them. However, we had been wanting a baby for so long that we were still so enthralled with the fact that we were pregnant so we did not let our worries pop our blissful bubbles until we received our amniocentesis results at 28 weeks.

That's when our world came crashing down.

Getting to grow, love and parent Saylor, was my life's honor. I feel so lucky to have been chosen as her mother. The connection she and I have is unlike any other. I still feel as close to her as I did when she was in my belly. It's funny because I remember saying I wish she could stay in my belly forever before I gave birth to her. She just seemed too happy and safe in there. I was so scared of what the outside world would bring to her. So many scary unknowns. But even post-delivery and post-death, I still feel her presence just as much as I always have. She is still very much a part of our current life and always will be.

Saylor and I shared so many special bonds and memories. One of my most cherished is the way we slept together. Because of her health conditions, she felt most comfortable at an incline to help with her extreme acid reflux and breathing issues. Lucky for my husband and I, we have an adjustable mattress frame that allows for such a thing. Because of this, and the

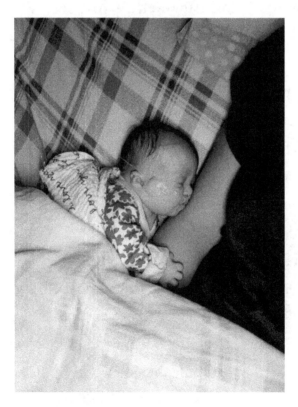

fact that she was most at peace while snuggling close to her parents, she slept in our King size tempurpedic bed with us every night. Despite our efforts to prop pillow partitions around her to avoid her rolling into unsafe positions, she always seemed to find a way to be close to me. I have dozens of photos of Saylor and I waking up in the morning in bed. I would snap a picture almost every morning to memorialize how cute she looked and so I could always remember how she would inch closer to me throughout the night just to wind up basically nose to nose. It's like she could sense or smell exactly where I was in the bed and maneuver her little body like an inchworm closer and closer to me until we were touching. There were so few things that seemed to truly console Saylor and my presence really seemed to be one and that made my momma heart so happy and proud. One of the positive outlooks on Saylor's short little life was the impact of love she was able to feel in just her year of existence (9 months pregnant and 3.5 months on earth). Saylor was able to feel more love in 3 months than some children get to experience in their whole lives.

Someone once explained the death of a child as, "you're always a lot closer to tears and never laugh quite as hard ever again." This I find to be very true. You are forever different after your child dies. No one really prepares you for the "after." The overwhelming grief is all the love you want to give but cannot. It bottles up in your soul, gathers up in the corner of your eyes and burns that hollow part of your chest. It has the ability to take your breath away and it's knowing that no matter how many tears you've cried, there's always a million more to spare. I'm certain you never get over the loss of your child because it's quite physically, emotionally, and spiritually impossible. You will always feel the raw emptiness that you eventually learn to coexist with. But I'm certain it changes you to the core.

I want to thank Saylor for the joy of being her earthly mother and forever momma in Heaven. I've never been more proud of anything in my entire life.

Saylor, being your mom is my most sacred journey–you are and always will be loved for eternity. I can't wait to see you again!

That is one thing that has helped more than anything else...knowing we will see her again. If we didn't have that and our faith, oh how lost we would be.

Resources:

KrabbeConnect:
Committed to pioneering a patient centered care model and strengthening groundbreaking research by engaging patients and caregivers with the Krabbe research community, to ensure the needs of Krabbe parents are being voiced. https://krabbeconnect.org
Email: info@krabbeconnect.org
Address: PO Box 254 Rosemount, MN 55068
Phone: 1-800-800-5509

Compassionate Friends:
Offers friendship, understanding, and hope to families grieving the death of a child at any age from any cause. With more than 600 chapters and more than 25 closed Facebook pages, it remains the largest self help bereavement support organization in the United States. Local chapters offer monthly, peer-to-peer support meetings. https://www.compassionatefriends.org

Hospice:

Care is for people who are nearing the end of life. The services are provided by a team of healthcare professionals who maximize comfort for a person who is terminally ill by reducing pain and addressing physical, psychological, social and spiritual needs.

Counseling:

Tips on finding a counselor who is a good fit :

- Find a counselor with training and experience in an area, like grief, infant loss, etc.
- Someone who is collaborative and tolerates questions about compatibility.
- Open to interviewing for a good fit.
- If it's a Pastor, there should be training in psychology or counseling.
- Experience doesn't always mean competency.
- The process of finding a counselor is not easy, and if it's not a good fit, don't fight it.
- You can find someone faith based (or not) depending on your preference.

Focus on good health:

- Exercise and fresh air are rejuvenating.
- A healthy diet will give your body energy to heal and grieve.
- Limit alcohol and drugs as they may numb for a short time, but they can make the situation worse.
- See your doctor if you feel you need help with medication. Antidepressants and/or sleep aids can help and may only be needed for a short time.
- Drink lots of water and try to get a good night's sleep.
- Instead of burying the pain, experience it and surround yourself with supportive friends. This is a time where YOU choose those with whom you want to spend time.
- Utilize music, journaling, or whatever you enjoy as you process your grief.
- We made stuffed bears and put Saylor's recorded heartbeat inside so we can listen to that forever.

"So we do not lose heart. Though our outer self is wasting away, our inner self is being renewed day by day. For this light momentary affliction is preparing us for an eternal weight of glory beyond all comparison, as we look not to the things that are seen but to the things that are unseen. For the things that are seen are transient, but the things that are unseen are eternal."

2 Corinthians 4:16-18

Printed in the USA
CPSIA information can be obtained
at www.ICGtesting.com
JSHW012355150923
48206JS00003B/13